7 STEP TO WEIGHT- LESS

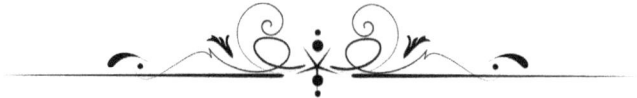

7-STEP TO WEIGHT-LESS

Or

How to Eat Chocolate, Drink
Alcohol & Still Love Your Mirror

Author

ZHENYA VERNON

CONTENTS

Foreword

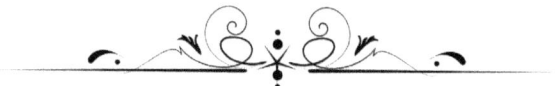

"I don't want my wrinkles taken away – I don't want to look like everyone else."

~ Jane Fonda

Why have you not been able to get the body shape of your dreams?

Have you ever thought about how much easier your everyday life would be if you had a better body, attracting more people and attained more goals? You might ask yourself: "Why haven't I achieved it yet? What *else* can I do to get the body shape I really want? Why are others happy with their bodies — am I *so* different?"

The truth is, other people are similar to you. It's not that you're less skilled, less attractive or less motivated than those whom you admire. They can carry their bodies with confidence, choose to wear the latest fashions, or proudly wear a bathing suit. *Finding the right balance between your lifestyle and physical shape doesn't depend on whether you are good enough or not.*

So...why do you still struggle?

Certain behaviors, thoughts or emotions have unconsciously been affecting how you look and feel.

You probably made several critical attempts and mistakes in managing, nourishing and developing your body.

You've read some articles and tried dieting. May be you had a personal trainer, but the results did not last? Most likely, you simply couldn't dive deeply into the subject to learn everything yourself because your field of expertise doesn't allow time for it?

You can't imagine reading fifty books to learn everything about health and fitness yourself?

The reality is you're possibly just trying to get sleep between assignments in a high-paced lifestyle instead of browsing the "health" section of a bookstore. Unless you plan to enroll yourself for a degree in nutrition or exercise science or permanently employ a trainer, read "7 STEP To Weight-Less" to attain your goal. It's specifically written to provide you with insight to the personal training process so that you don't have to spend more money on random diets, pills and inefficient exercise routines.

Remember, that...

ALL successful training programs are based on universal principles of anatomy and physiology, which are NOT subject to change, ever. Underlying science and common sense will determine the structure of your own plans.

This book contains a range of fitness knowledge that nutritionists and exercise coaches around the world learn BEFORE they educate others. I simply consolidated the best information available from studies, mentors and from numerous health top events around the world. Included are my personal practical experiences too, as I have been involved for moreover then 20 years in different amateur and professional activities, from figure skating to body shaping competitions, so I maintain excellent physical shape to present day.

After reading this book, you may stop relying on what works for your friends and relatives, and finally make your own decisions about what works best for your own physique. It will guide you to make the right choice that works specifically for *you*.

Enjoy!

STEP 1. Are You Ready?

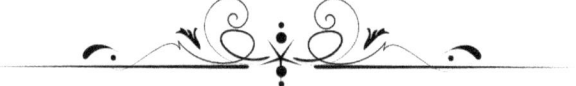

"We often have courage, praise an effort but only results deserve true reward."

~ Author

There are certain excuses people create that hinder themselves from eating well or exercising regularly. They may be unaware of the benefits, or simply believe they have no "time" to train.

Some people follow new diet plans and/or training programs that are too long or too complicated, and don't achieve promised results for their investments.

Some programs may promote deprivation, even injury, or require excessive time, unusual equipment, or the environment itself can be intimidating.

Research shows that most common reason that people give up on dieting or their training effort is "the perception of required time versus reality to achieve the expected result."

Before embarking on a new plan or routine, you probably asked yourself: *What if I fail? What if people laugh at me? What if I get hurt?* Begin by saying: "I *will* succeed. It *will* work and if I make a mistake, it will be a great learning experience that others (and I) will be proud of the effort."

Do you believe with certainty that being fit is attainable for the rest of your life? Can you imagine being powerfully committed to your most important health and fitness goal? And that means ***never, never, never give up***?

Sure you do! To go full speed ahead...

All you need is a program that will be:

- Time efficient and interesting
- Achievable and realistic
- Science-based and enjoyable
- And...part of your routine for the rest of your life

After your personal health and fitness goals are visualized, then you are ready to embark on an action plan set to achieve them.

Next, you will go through *five stages of change* to incorporate these new habits into your life. You may be a beginner, relatively fit, or an athlete with specific sporting or social events to prepare for with unique goals and timelines. Regardless of your purpose, there are **five major stages of change** you will go through before the "new pattern" will be easy enough to become "routine" in your everyday life. Here they are:

1. **Pre-contemplation stage**: I am not changing my diet/exercise and not intending to.
2. **Contemplation stage**: I am not changing my diet/exercise but intend to soon.
3. **Preparation stage**: I am making some changes, but I'm not fully committed.
4. **Action stage**: I have achieved a regular change for less than three months.
5. **Maintenance**: I am following all changes in my diet/exercise for over three months.

Your readiness for *change* will depend on your current stage of motivation for achieving your health and fitness goals. Let's define at which stage are you in at the moment.

Incidentally, most of people are at the *contemplation stage*, as they are "intending" to start their new weight loss or muscle gain regimen "soon."

Like most people, you probably won't be psychologically ready to jump stages, even after creating an ideal, totally self-managed eating plan or exercising program. That simply won't serve you long term.

So...what to do?

First, become *passionate* about your goal. Learn about the benefits of changing your activity levels, whether you're trying to lose fat or to build strength.

You must believe that new behavior is a worthwhile effort. The "pros" for adopting it outweigh the "cons" of change.

For example, creating time to go to the gym after work to lose weight should counter the cons of not being able to have a chat with friends after work, or watching your favorite shows on the couch.

You must believe in yourself *first*, and obliterate the notion that you can't perform a task successfully when it comes to your personal health or body shape.

At the end of the day, a better body creates healthy self-esteem, leading to greater career and relationship success.

Even more: you will be able to confidently wear your swimsuit on a beach. It won't happen overnight, but with patience, it **will** happen.

Fitness professionals can assist you with support, handouts and information about the constant benefits of healthy nutrition and physical activity.

But you won't be alone if you choose not to have a trainer...

Your questions must be answered: *How often should I eat and/or train? How much? How hard? How long my training session should last? What exactly to do to achieve my goal?* Obviously, how long it will take will depend on your enthusiasm for progress.

Believe me, even *you* inspire me to look good, that is, if you choose to follow my advice using this book. My hope is that you get better results then I did, and keep them over a lifetime.

Personally, I live up to my own standards to remain a physical role model in the eyes of friends, colleagues, partner, and even strangers...and I love turning heads too!

Now, let's define your preferred style of learning to understand your fastest way to a new "change":

Are you **auditory?** Do you learn by listening to recorded information/explanations over and over again? Do you prefer to tell to somebody as to hear it again and again? Can you listen to a song, act it out, or teach something to those who will listen?

Maybe you are **visual?** Do you learn by watching somebody else perform an example? Do you prefer seeing pictures, demonstrations, videos, reading and seeing words?

Do you love to touch tangible things, and are **kinesthetic?** Do you learn by doing something, like creating a model, designs, touching, feeling moods, practicing on somebody else?

HINT: your mind only remembers images. That's why you forget names but never a face. The other two most powerful ways to remember are smell and taste. You can tell because good food always smells...*good*.

To wrap it up: think about your body how it looks like right now...and draw an invisible line to how you want it to look. Make sure you have a *deadline* for the project. Just as you would in a business model of decision-making, you will be going through the following steps:

1. Get as many facts as possible.
2. Analyze the facts.
3. What is the worst-case scenario?
4. What is ideal scenario?
5. What is one thing you can do to avoid the worst circumstance?
6. Act, and don't look back.
7. If things are not working out, stop and start again, going back to step ONE.

Finally, learn to *accept* how you look or feel right now. Can you see how much work you will have to do to get from where are you now to where you would like to be?

Admit to yourself that making "excuses" for not changing, or "blaming" your social environment, or even being in "denial" that you need a change and you think you don't...will make your effort unsuccessful, unrewarding and may sabotage the results.

See yourself fit, healthy, and never doubt your success!

Step 2. Think 'Weight-Less'.

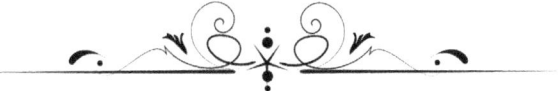

"In the absence of clearly-defined goals we become strangely loyal to performing daily trivia until ultimately we become enslaved by it."

~ Robert Heinlein

You are reading this because you want to increase the quality and length of your life.

This might include an initial consultation with a fitness or health professional to identify your own personal health and fitness goals, or what motivates you to want to make a change.

Another task is to access your needs, abilities and limitations to determine whether or not you are ready for the change you want. A professional would be able to help determine if your goals are in line with realistic expectations.

Here are some of the top reasons why people want a change:

- Weight loss or fat loss

- Changing body shape or tone

- To fit into latest designer outfits

- To get more energy and feel better

- To increase fitness and quality of life

During your first consultation with a fitness professional, you may be asked questions as to "why", "where", and by "when" would you want to have a change in your body shape or general fitness to get and keep the body shape you want.

Think about how successful would you feel if you achieve it? How frustrated would it make you if you didn't? If you continue on your regular routine, would you achieve your goal? What are you prepared to do, or to give up to achieve it?

What are the barriers holding you back from taking steps to change your exercise and eating patterns?

Is there is something or someone who you think may help?

The most popular reason to kick start exercise is an upcoming *event*: reaching a goal associated with the Big Day. A "Big Day" can be a wedding, vacation, marathon, mountain climbing or even a date with that special someone.
However, planning for such a special occasion can sometimes cloud other aspects of our health.
One should consider other habits, including alcohol consumption, smoking, sleep deprivation, or stress that leads to heartburn/indigestion and fatigue.

Monitor any obstacles that might affect your fitness goals. Making an "Event Planning Checklist" will help you find the success you aim for.

You will need *structured strategies* to become involved with the process quickly. It is good to write down your plan's decisions, so that you will feel double responsibility to follow programs and you'll be more likely to reach your goals.

17

F Y I

Question: What is sufficient physical activity for a healthy, fit body?

Answer: Average thirty minutes of moderate intensity exercise four to five days a week. A total of 150 minutes of moderate activity per week is enough to achieve health benefits. The best results are achieved in short sessions ranging from ten to thirty minutes, during a brisk walk, swimming, tennis, cycling, jogging, or rowing.

The good news is that when you maintain your achieved condition, you can exercise even less to keep the same result. Yay! No one said that starting up is easy. Just compare it to looking for a new job in a country you just landed and hardly speak the language!

If you weren't doing any physical activity at all, you would be classified as "sedentary." These types struggle to jog for even two minutes. Certainly, you want to have better results than that.

Don't forget that domestic activity (like gardening or cleaning house) and work activity also contribute to overall physical activity.

So, as long as your keeping up around the home or work, things aren't that bad!

Let's bring some science into the equation: scientists use four major principles for your new, customized dieting or exercise routine.

They include **frequency**, **intensity**, **time** and **type** of an exercise to determine your working and leisure lifestyle patterns.

You should always consult a health professional to examine your cardiovascular risk. They can assess how "fit" you are to participate in any activity and if you require special medical instructions.

They will consider your sleep, work and social patterns, any muscle issues, painful conditions you might have, eating disorders or food allergies. These all have a huge impact on how to design your most efficient, safe and effective program.

Fitness tests are a *must*. They provide valuable progress regarding your improvement and results. This will ensure you are progressing toward your goals. Tests are usually repeated at least every 12 weeks to determine if you need to re-valuate your goals. Basic tests include resting heart rate, resting blood pressure, flexibility (sit and reach), and waist circumference: excessive abdominal fat may increase heart disease risk in men with a measurement of over 94 cm, and 80 cm in women.

One more time... the benefits of being fit:

- Improved and stronger heart muscle and breathing rate

- More lean body mass and less body fat

- Improved overall strength and endurance

- Flexibility, lower heart rate, lower blood pressure

- Reduced blood cholesterol

- Reduced chance of coronary heart disease

- Greater chance of surviving heart attack

- Improved appearance, greater perception of body image

- Reduced chance of injury, improved performance

- Resistance to fatigue, higher energy levels, less stress

- Better sex and enhanced body ability to enjoy leisure

- Improved self-worth, quality of life, coping skills

- Sense of well-being, enhanced recovery from work

- Delay in aging process

- Acceptance of personal limitations

  ...And much, much more benefits await if you can enroll into a new lifetime eating plan and/or exercise program to create positive, long term effects on your health and fitness.

See you fit, healthy and never without support!

Step 3. Getting H.E.L.P.

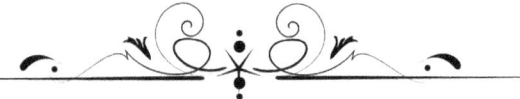

"We should look for someone to eat and drink with before looking for something to eat and drink."

~ EPICURUS

You might need real **H.E.L.P.** to get where you want to be. What is that, you really ask??

"H" – *Healthy*...
"E" – *Eating*...
"L" – *Lifestyle*...
"P" – *Plan*...

When is a good time to start with **H.E.L.P.?**

RIGHT NOW**...**

But don't panic! It takes a little bit of time to understand your personal relationship with food before you go any further.

Begin this process by identifying your likes, dislikes, preferences and emotions about food before you venture into a costly nutrition consultation with a specialist.

Here is a list of questions to ask yourself:

- What do you *like* to eat?

- Which foods are most frequently in your fridge?

- What would you prefer not to or *wouldn't* eat?

- When (and why) do you normally eat?

- How do you feel about deprivation and how it affects your body shape?

- Are you mostly motivated to eat "healthy" food that gives you energy, strength, and a well performing body?

Remember that eating plans that work for someone else will be irrelevant for YOU. There are so many choices to eat healthy these days with all the diets around.

Have you ever wondered what the most attractive people do for their eating plans?

"Normal eating" is different for everyone. However, it is NOT normal to count calories or weigh food. It is NOT normal to eat the same amount of food every day. It is NOT normal to be rigid by limiting food choices.

It is absolutely NORMAL to overeat *occasionally*, to eat at least three times a day, to avoid eating certain types of food, to have fluctuations in appetite or crave certain "addictive" foods due to hormonal or emotional imbalances.

Food is one of the greatest pleasures in life. No one should eat the foods they dislike, just because they are considered "healthy."

Make an effort to satisfy your palate by making a weekly food checklist. Contact me to send you basic templates to track your true preferences, so that you can make a realistic eating plan to achieve your goal.

Your lifestyle may be not match that of the current Mr. Olympia or celebrities that share their "secrets" of fat loss and belly reduction in the latest issue of "Woman's Weekly," so don't fall into the trap of following their footsteps. Most likely, they're paying a team of specialists that monitor their every step!

Different occupations require appropriate dietary needs. Busy massage therapists or personal trainers may feel hungry every two to three hours versus an office worker that is sitting down at a desk or during endless business meetings.

If you are a surgeon performing laparoscopies or hip and knee replacements, you probably can't stop and take a quality food break. Occupations like lawyers or dentists too can be busy for up to eight hours a day, making it difficult to spare a minute to put together a whole-grain bread toast spread with low-fat cream cheese for a quick energy fix snack.

Perhaps you watched the documentary, "FOOD," by Michael Moore, and became not so fond of read meat that you became a vegetarian. If so, it could be a challenge for you to follow what health professionals typically advise: to increase your iron intake from animal products, thus rejuvenating your red blood cells?

Emotional challenges to eating plans can be in the form of eating disorders.

If allowed to go to extremes, they can negatively affect the quality of your life, leading to poor health, cancer, and even death. Emotional eaters are "controlled by food." Do you live to eat, or eat to live? In normal circumstances, eating should not be triggered by your mood.

There are also short-term eating conditions known as "Anorexia Nervosa," or "Bulimia Nervosa," which are a more typical disorder for women.

"Megarexia" or a mental condition where one perceives one's body as too thin and desires to be larger, mainly affects the male population.

Some young men see their body shape as "too small" and become obsessed with eating and exercising: they often use or abuse supplements to build their physique and never feel big enough. "Obesity" and "binge eating" strongly affect both sexes with a rate of at least 45% of women, and 60% of men. This is especially true in economically developed societies like USA, Australia, UK, and parts of Spain and Italy, where food is abundant and simply "everywhere."

The best diet plans are:

- Enjoyable and scientifically based
- Realistic and time efficient
- Achievable and something you can stick with for the rest of your life

Whenever you discover a "new diet" fad online, in a published book or magazine, apply the principles above to estimate the "ease" of such diet alternatives for yourself.

Whatever is the best way for you to eat to your goal will be a personal choice. Whether it's to lose weight, tone up, increase your sporting performance, to prepare for marathon, or to monitor your intake of fats, protein and carbohydrates, the desired result is found through a generic formula of the *World Science of Weight Loss*:

ENERGY "IN" < ENERGY "OUT"

In essence, if you consume less food and drinks than what your body is using through movement for maintaining optimal temperature, the body starts to use stored fat to burn energy.

That means you will lose weight!

The opposite happens if you desire muscle mass gain: *ENERGY "IN" > ENERGY "OUT"*.

From the nutrition point of view, the body doesn't know the difference between "good" and "bad" foods you consume.

It doesn't care how excess energy ended up there. The body only counts "calories." Just as a banker won't ask you where your money is coming from, so long as you keep depositing it in their account with a positive balance.

But all things considered, you wouldn't want to sacrifice your *health*, would you?

In case you missed the basic food group courses, here are the rules of eating: Healthy Food Pyramid.

This great "triangle" has been published in more then 100,000 books, so you can trust it is a *safe* guide.

Food Guide Pyramid
A Guide to Daily Food Choices

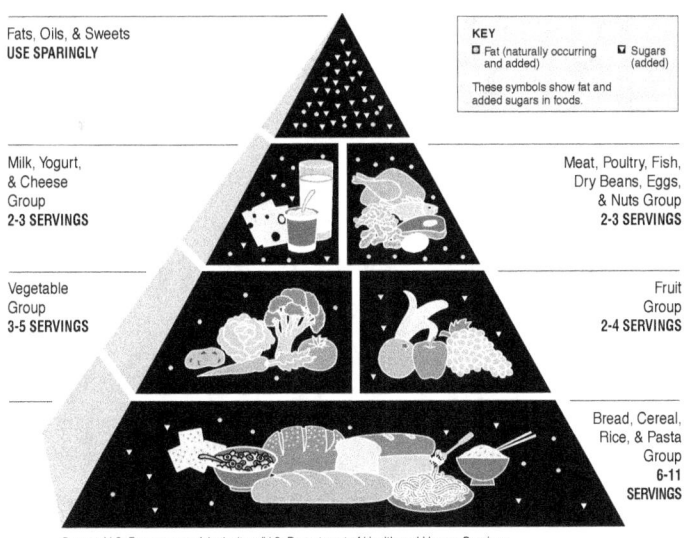

Source: U.S. Department of Agriculture/U.S. Department of Health and Human Services

The most effective and essential strategy to design your H.E.L.P. (Healthy Eating Lifestyle Plan) is to include enjoyable and realistic choices that you can stick to for the rest of your life.

Looking further into your diet plan, you'll need to learn know more about food labeling and nutritional contents. This will help determine the vitamins, minerals, and enzymes, and how much of each you will need.

You'll be able to make smart choices as opposed to "junk food," especially when you aren't familiar with a culinary cuisine.

You can then master the skill of dieting and avoid the crazy, vicious yo-yo cycles most dieters go through, including myself in a recent past.

Most of the popular "detox" diets are based on calorie restriction (deprivation) and may feel like you're starving. Unfortunately, the weight you lose in a few days may not even be fat but from water and muscle tissue.

Muscle tissue loss slows down your metabolic rate, thus slowing down fat-burning rate simultaneously. Hence, once you are back on your usual, non-diet routine, you will regain the weight you lost.

Unless you choose to continue depriving yourself, massive calorie cutbacks mean less energy, leading to a dysfunctional affect on all levels of your wellbeing. When you suddenly cut back food portions, you not only feel tired but also your body shifts into "starvation" mode.

The calorie-burning process slows down as the body tries to hold onto stored fat (that was there in case of such an emergency, assuring a supply of energy when needed).

Our fat cells may "shrink" in size, but remain vulnerable to gaining back everything they lost once your "diet" is finished. This is a life preservation mechanism, genetically built-in to save and increase fat-producing cells at times of starvation.

Conclusion: while trying to lose fat, you will actually

increase your chance of gaining weight after your diet is over.

So it's best to eat foods that fly and move "off the ground," move your body more, and for goodness sake, NEVER DIET!!

To wrap it up, here are a few replacement tips on "how to turn fat into skinny meals" (and don't be afraid to ask about it in restaurants, too):

- Cream… replace with low-fat yogurt
- Milk… substitute full cream milk for ½ or skim milk
- Baking… use foil and lemon juice, and bake meats in the oven instead of deep-frying
- Cakes… replace butter or oil with orange juice; use two egg whites rather than one whole egg
- Frying food… use non-stick pan or use a brush or cooking spray to add oil rather then pouring it
- Cream cheese… replace with cottage cheese wetted with milk or yogurt
- Stewing or sautéing… use water or soup stock to simmer instead of adding oil

See you fit, healthy and never hungry!

Step 4. Stay erect.

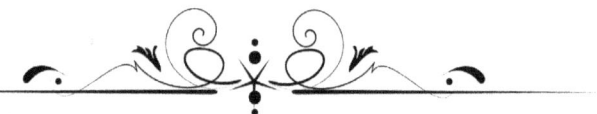

"Women have a wonderful instinct about things. They can discover everything except the obvious."

~ Oscar Wilde

To minimize the risk of injury, your program shall fit your lifestyle, rather than changing your lifestyle to fit the program.

According to the rules of strength training and exercise progression when you ready to climb onto a next level, try to answer the following questions during your program, or at least start thinking about it:

- Is a chosen exercise *safe* and functional based on your anatomy?
- Is it *appropriate* for how you move on a daily basis?
- Is it *beneficial* to you, and do you enjoy doing it?
- Is there is a *better* exercise you could do to meet your goal faster?

Choose exercises that enhance staying erect, and avoid any that would negatively affect your posture.

Fitness professionals can assist you in finding the correct routine while conducting fitness tests.

So, what are your goals at this point?

- **POSTURE**: If you exercise with poor posture, you will wear your tendons and joints out. Just like when you start learning anything for the first time, especially with use of equipment, it is advisable to select a "device" that is easy to operate and doesn't require "high performance." Start with a machine-based gym routine that has a lower degree of complexity. It should be easy to manage compared to free weight exercises.

- **RANGE OF MOVEMENT**: During a training routine, your joints should have pain-free and safe movement. To work out painlessly, you usually can go outside of your perception of how much you can really do. So, don't be afraid to try a bit harder. It will be more effective to strive to lift or push weight beyond your comfort zone, especially in squat and chest exercises with minimal up-down movement. True range of movement is often similar to your daily routine during work or free time activities.

- **STABILITY**: Uncontrolled movements, such as falling over, leaning, applying uneven, heavy or incorrect forces on the muscles, bones and other structures of your musculoskeletal system may cause premature wear of your joints and soft tissues. The result could be injury and/or dislocations. Make sure to keep your posture erect while walking, running or lifting something considerably heavy from the ground.

- **PERFORMANCE**: Most of us learn to move without losing stability of our neck, scapula, shoulder, lower back, hips and knee joints. If you keep that stability in mind, you may increase the weight or load while doing your favorite strength training, and increase intensity of the cardio training exercises. *Remember*: without correct posture, range of movement, and stability, you can't have a good performance!

Did you know, that most of people go straight to step four (performance), doing a lot of complex exercises without first mastering the techniques of the preceding steps. As a result, injuries can occur and a rehabilitation program may be prescribed instead!

Posture is the foremost thing you should be concerned with.

Not only will it hide or show your natural beauty, but also it reflects how you carry yourself through your walking pattern.

There are also certain conditions that may lead to postural abnormalities, including birth defects, carrying excessive weight, repetitive occupations and sporting activities, muscle imbalances, or differences in the length of one's legs.

Those imbalances place excessive stress on joints, muscles, and ligaments, and can lead to a painful degeneration of one's physique.

So, how do you start?

Undress and look at your body in a mirror. Make self-examination to determine whether you have a good posture, or if it is being affected by slouching in the same position.

True fitness professional can measure the length of your muscle to find your realistic abilities and strengths. That is an essential part of gathering knowledge to prescribe correct exercise program.

Why?

Well, most exercises are designed to stretch short muscles or to strengthen weak muscles. This, in turn, will help you know what your muscles are capable of, and their ability to provide stability of your joints for correct posture and support.

It's imperative to be aware about your personal limitations during a thorough testing, so that the correct exercise technique can be prescribed and maintained.

Do you may have one or combination of postural imbalances?

- **Scoliosis**: abnormal sideways curvature of the spine ('s' shape)
- **Kyphosis**: excessive curvature of the thoracic spine, resulting in a "hunch-back" posture development
- **Lordosis**: exaggerated curvature in lumbar spine, or "sway-back"
- **Flat Back**: a lack of curvature in the lumbar spine
- **Rounded Shoulders**: mild-case kyphosis, scapulae sticks out
- **Forward Neck**: excessively protruding neck, or "poke chin"
- **Flat Neck**: excessive flat upper back, or "military posture"

- **Genu Varum**: outward-curving of the legs (bow), resulting in a gap between knees while standing
- **Genu Valgum**: inward-curving of the legs (knock-knees), resulting in a gap between feet when the knees are in contact
- **Foot Pronation**: turning the feet outward excessively

Did you recognize any of those forms of poor posture in the mirror?

Good luck, and see you fit, healthy and poised for greatness!

Step 5. Jumping High.

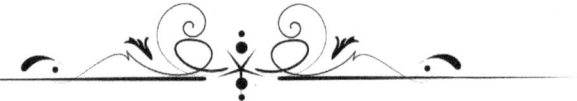

"Two things are bad for the heart-- running up stairs and running down people."
~ Bernard M. Baruch

There are few basic activity options to help lose body fat once you've determined your eating plans. Cardiovascular training is the next step up, where *time commitment* would be the key to success.

The purpose of aerobic training is to enhance "endurance." You have many choices: skipping rope, climbing stairs, boxing, bicycling, treadmill, stepper, skiers and rowers, cross-training, rowing, power walking and running.

All of these activities will decrease the intensity of lactic acid being dispersed over time. That means your body will tire "slower," giving you more energy for life!

How do you start, and what is "enough?"

One hundred minutes a week of planned aerobic or cardio movement is sufficient in maintaining healthy heart and lungs.

Ideally, you can spread those 100 minutes in sets of time periods: 2 sessions at 50 minutes, or 3 at 33, 4 at 25, 5 at 20, and even 20 at 5.

Most people choose 20 minutes a day as a regular "must do" activity, so it accommodates to their lifestyle. Regardless of the combination, all time-sets produce the same health benefits as long as the minimum time has been covered throughout the week.

Five simple steps to start:

1. Do an activity.
2. Aim for 100 minutes a week.
3. Do something every day.
4. Aim to do the same amount in less time.
5. Choose alternative activities or do the same differently.

Your professionally designed cardio program would consist of:

1. Warm up (preparation phase)
2. Workout (conditioning phase)
3. Cool down (recovery phase)
4. Recovery (adaptation phase)

Most conditioning specialists suggest exercising at least three days a week, with *no more* then two days between workouts to keep body fat at optimal levels.

For "sedentary" people, or beginners, at least three days of rest between sessions is recommended, especially if they choose high-impact running activity.

Why?

Muscles need time to adapt to hard movement to avoid fatigue, injury or muscle soreness.

The American College of Sports Medicine (ACSM) suggests that people with difficulties performing every day should try activities such as getting up from a chair or walking to get the benefit from sessions of 3 to 5 minutes spread throughout the day.

As fitness improves, 20 minute sessions for 3 to 5 days a week are allowed, moving toward 30 minute sessions of moderate intensity during most days of the week.

If you are prepared to work out as hard and long as possible, you may achieve an athletic level of performance in preparation for a marathon or other event - just like a true fitness professional.

After about six weeks, your program will be moved to a higher level, and the elements will include:

- Modes of training (strength, flexibility, endurance)
- Structure and techniques (full body, circuit)
- Training frequency
- Warm up and stretching
- Exercise selection
- Number of sets and repetitions
- Speed of movement
- Recovery

See you fit, healthy, and never out of breath!

Step 6. Take On A Heavy Duty.

"Intensity builds immensity."

~ Kevin Levrone

The next step is to incorporate an *exercise program* into your lifestyle. It may be in a gym, circuit, outdoors, a field, track or even hotel or office environment.

Regardless of your fitness level or where you are, this program will contain three major components of fitness:

1. **Strength** (muscular strength)

2. **Stamina** (cardiovascular fitness)

3. **Suppleness** (flexibility)

You will learn to find a balance between those three important factors. Gradually, you will combine some extra work for agility, power, joint stability and coordination for complete body health.

Every single exercise will consist of these parts:

- **Frequency** (how often)

- **Intensity** (how hard)

- **Type** (walk, jog, swim, massage)

- **Time** (how long)

You will learn ***progressive overload*** concept: the continual increase in load applied to the body, as you adapt to the previous impact.

You will see improvement in overall performance during the ***super-compensation process***, explained later, how well you can progress once you recover from training: initially, you will experience exhaustion, but your stamina will become stronger with time.

You will have more **power**, which is measured how quickly you able to lift the same barbell as opposed to another person who lifts it in a longer period of time (0,5 sec vs. 1 sec).

Strength will determine how much force your muscle group can exert against resistance (weights, cables, body weight) in one (maximal) movement called "contraction," called by exercise scientists as "1RM".

Your training session will consist of four sequential phases:

1.   **Preparation phase** (general warm up). This phase psychologically prepares the body for an exercise, while reducing risk of injury. You want a gradual increase in muscle temperature, elasticity, heart rate, oxygen supply, release of synovial fluid to lubricate joints and neural transmission.

    You can choose from a massage, saunas, spas, tracksuits, and hot water bottles to light cardio, such as walking, jogging, bike riding and rowing.

    Specific warm-up performed after the general preparation include exercises related to your fitness goal, such as push-ups and light weight warm-up sets, "suicide runs" or anything you enjoy doing.

2.   **Conditioning phase** (workout) will include either muscle work or aerobic exercises, depending what's on your agenda. A selection of exercises will determine the result you want to achieve.
This is where you will be losing the most weight, your muscles become stronger and endurance levels will boost your energy for life.

3.   **Cool down phase** is a recovery stage for tapering-off after your main working-out effort. Continued, low intensity movement within five or fewer minutes will decrease your heart rate.

This helps to avoid blood pooling, and slows down breathing. It prepares you for stretching and recovery.

4.   **Adaptation phase** or "recovery." Genetics, lifestyle, occupational stressors, sleep, nutrition and medication will affect how quickly you recover from the session.

The frequency of your training will depend on how quickly you and your body systems fatigue and recover on neuromuscular, hormonal and "mental" levels to be ready for your next work out.

Big questions must be answered:

• How short can my program be?
• How fast can I get results if I spend less time in a gym?
• How many sessions per week will produce

optimal results?
- How many sets or repetitions will bring the best results?

Get used to words like *repetitions, rest intervals, reversibility, sets and speed of movement, velocity, training volume, training stimulus, adaptation and threshold.*

Always monitor your heart rate during training as a way to track your intended goal.

You *maximal heart rate* will be 220 minus your age. Your *ideal heart rate* that you normally exercise with will be different, depending on your training goal and fitness level.

To reach faster and better results, you must know how to calculate workout intensity depending on the body shape you want to achieve.

Did you know there are scientifically based principles of optimal gains in muscle strength?

Or that size can be achieved in a very short period of time in brief sessions?

Isn't one of your goals to be able to spend less time but achieve more?

Your program may include **stretching** to improve your ***balance*** – to maintain equilibrium while your body is stationary or moving.

Better ***flexibility*** will increase range of movement of muscles through work on a specific joint.

Cardiovascular fitness, such as aerobics, running or walking over two minutes at a time will help the heart and blood vessels as well as the respiratory system to supply more oxygen to working muscles while removing metabolic wastes (lactate, CO_2). You will feel more energy and lose fat even faster.

You may want to dance and move fast, as you work on your ability to combine movement in different body parts over a period of time – *coordination and mobility.*

Increased ability to change the direction of the body in space rapidly will enhance *agility*.

Endurance is important as your muscles may contract longer against given resistance in certain period of time You may burn even more fat and become fitter in no time while lasting longer before getting tired.

See you fit, healthy and full of energy!

Step 7. The Art Of Lazy.

"Hard work never killed anybody, but why take a chance?"

~ Edgar Bergen

Putting together fitness routine and fitting into a week is the most difficult part for many people. It's the main reason why you may not be able to manage an "all-around" fitness method to your fat loss.

Remember that you've earned the recovery period when you're really tired, not just because a bed is there.

Remember, that you deserve to eat when you are physically hungry, not because you have easy access to food.

Basic things like using stairs instead of an elevator, walking instead of a short drive, occasionally moving around your office instead of sitting for lengthy periods, parking *intentionally* farther are non-negotiable standards to live by.

Why is recovery is needed?

The golden rule is, "safety first," so a preferred program won't hurt you.

However, you may experience muscle soreness post-exercise within 48 hours after unaccustomed exercise. It results from tiny tears in muscle tissue through nerve endings, causing a painful sensation.

It is exacerbated by a workout that includes unusual types of contractions. This is absolutely normal. "No pain; no gain."

If your muscles still feel "spent," get a sports massage, or use an icepack on sore areas. Simple walks, stretching routines, or taking vitamins C and E, (from melons, berries, nuts, green vegetables and oils) can also alleviate soreness.

Try to avoid over the counter drugs, like popular "Ibuprofen," as its prolonged use may result in liver damage and reduce your body's ability to fight inflammation.

Sleep well!

A lack of a rest reduces a body's ability to produce glucose.

Ways to compensate are with warm showers, mid-day naps, listening to music, watching movies.

Massages and stretching are traditionally the best ways to recover after a session.

Tips to remember:

- Don't stretch before gym work or for 3 to 4 hours afterwards. Light stretching in your warm ups and cool downs are preferable.

- Be sure you are prepared to give 100% effort into each training, cardio, or weight session. Know what you will need to do afterward.

- Food is important. Be sure to have a supply of healthy snacks for before and after training.

- Have one day to completely rest. We can help you choose when you're creating the right training plan *for you*.

- Underlying science and common sense will determine the structure of your routines.

And, again...all programs must be based on *universal principles of anatomy and physiology*. These are NOT subject to change.

At last, overtraining is the main reason people get frustrated and end up quitting.

Some programs take too long, require too much work, are not hard enough, or follow incorrect techniques.

Your goal will be to find a balance between intensity and recovery to enjoy what you're doing - without struggling through it.

See you fit, healthy and never tired!

Bonus Tips.

"Knowledge comes, but wisdom lingers."

~ Alfred Lord Tennyson

*There are tried and true strategies for keeping you focused on **what works best** for your weight management:*

1. **EAT AND DRINK LESS CALORIES** – cutting back on the total amount of calories you consume is a winning strategy for weight loss. Target high-calorie, fatty and sugary foods first and cut back on alcohol. These dietary changes create the energy windfall that helps you to burn and reduce body fat.

2. **BURN MORE CALORIES** – the more you move your body every day, the more calories you'll burn up, which helps to create an even greater surge of energy. More daily movements, walking, and some strength training provide the best activity combinations.

3. **MANAGE YOUR APPETITE** – limit your portion sizes and avoid the habit of overeating. Choose foods that are filling and not fattening, like lean protein, salads, fruits and vegetables. Wholegrain products are good, too.

4. **KNOW YOUR EATING TRIGGERS** – identifying the people, places or thoughts that trigger you to overeat or to choose high calorie foods will allow you to plan alternatives and deal with situations that tend to trip you up. Surround yourself with other good influences.

5. **MONITOR YOUR PROGRESS** – track changes

to your diet and exercise routine to raise your awareness and keep you on the path to success.

6. **BUILD YOUR OWN SUPPORT NETWORK –** enlist family, friends or workmates to encourage and support you. You might even make a "biggest loser" challenge.

7. **GET PROFESSIONAL ADVICE** – use a weight loss adviser to share good information, tips and strategies to keep you focused and motivated.

8. **PERSONALISE YOUR PROGRAM** – as you progress, keep the diet strategies that work for you and ditch any that don't.

9. **CHOOSE TO LOSE THE CONFUSION** – make it your policy to critically filter the useless and distracting diet information you hear.

10. **BE FLEXIBLE** – allow yourself to have slip-ups and try not to let them become major setbacks. Lasting results come from a healthy attitude.

...AND...ARE YOU READY FOR SOMETHING MORE?

If you made it to the last chapter and absorbed all the information, I believe you've got an inspiration to start getting the body shape you want and deserve.

"If someone else got it – you can achieve it, too."
You already know what you need to get started.

You are already equipped with the tools at your disposal to get from where are you now to where you want to be.

All you need to do is to empower yourself in pursuing your very own, number one "health and fitness ideal" till you excel, and whether you have personal trainer or not. *"You do not live to eat or to move - you eat and move to live longer, healthier and happier."*

Balancing your physical health will automatically enhance your social (body image), mental (self-esteem), sexual (libido) and even career opportunities.

To start, you may need help to re-create your vision, to re-evaluate your health objectives or simply stay focused on your current number one "health and fitness goal" to assure your success.

The excerpt was written for you to make up your mind about what approach you choose to obtaining your goal BEFORE you start training!

Good Luck.

Zhenya.

www.ingramcontent.com/pod-product-compliance
Lightning Source LLC
Chambersburg PA
CBHW071330310526
45789CB00017B/2174